The Teenage Boy's guide to sexuality

A straight talking, guy to guy booklet on everything a teenage boy needs to know about his body.

The teenage boy's guide to sexuality

Copyright © 2018 by Tim Owen

ISBN: 978-1981746842

Teenage boys guide to sexuality

Teenage boys guide to sexuality

Dear parents,

I am male, plus have two teenage sons of my own and so I understand the unspoken fears and concerns that teenage boys have about sex and their bodies.

Most schools today have some form of sex-ed classes, but these cover the basic logistics and working of the sex organs in the context of coitus, seldom dealing with concerns of a more personal nature.

Moms, especially, like to cling to the notion that their little boys will be sweet and innocent into their twenties. It's difficult to think of them as sexual beings because that means they are growing up, and quite naturally, separating from you.

The fact is, they *are* growing up and they *are* becoming sexual beings. Too often, our own guilt, baggage, history or lack of willingness to let our sons go affects how we interact with them on the subject.

If you, like me, fall into that category of parent, then we have two choices here: create another generation of sexually dysfunctional people who will have issues around sex for their entire lives, or get over ourselves and give our sons the gift our parents denied us: unconditionally happy and healthy sex lives, and thereby, happy and stable relationships.

Mom's, there is something you need to know: your teenage sons masturbate. Yes, they do. It's *normal* and it's *healthy*. The possibility that your son does not masturbate is 0. If dad is with you, ask him. (http://www.healthystrokes.com/young.html)

Making a big deal of it or speaking of it as a shameful or sinful act is going to affect your son's perception of himself, and sex, for the rest of his life.

This often produces adults who either have great difficulty in maintaining relationships, are promiscuous or develop a porn addiction because it's safer than dating another sexual human being.

Masturbation is, in fact, *not* condemned in the bible, if that is the source of your opinion on the matter – read my chapter on it for clarity on this point.

Another thing you need to know is that when boys talk to each other, they don't use prissy words like masturbate and penis, they use *wank* and *cock*, or *dick*. These are *not* rude words, they are simply everyday guy-slang to replace medical terms. Accept these words as normal, and you remove the "naughtiness" and stigma around them as they become natural ways to describe an activity and a body part. If you find them offensive, remember that that stems from *your* conditioning, and *not* the view that you should be imparting to your sons.

On that note, it's time to decide if you are going to buy this book for your son, thereby letting him know that, a) you now know that he masturbates and that it's okay, and b) that you truly want him to grow up to be sexually confident and at ease with his body, and his sexuality, *whatever form it takes.*

One last thing: I am writing this book for our

sons, not for us parents, and so I am going to speak *their* language. I'm going to talk about wanking, cumming and cocks. If they want to know about masturbation and penises, they'll read a medical journal.

Thank you

Tim

Hello

Who should be reading this booklet?

Well, you've opened it so that means you have a normal and healthy interest and curiosity about sex and your body, so *you* should be reading it. This is not a clinical, dusty old medical journal full of terms like *penis, masturbation and ejaculation;* that's for the classroom, or to put you to sleep when you're suffering from insomnia.

We, as guys, talk about dicks, cocks,

jerking off, wanking and cumming; you probably know this already. I am talking to you as one guy to another, so let's talk in a language we both understand. I'll also be using many common terms, phrases and slang, in *italics* so you can pick them up easily.

Did that shock you? It may have; many elements of society make sex out to be a shameful, clinical act used primarily for reproduction. It's not. It's fun and healthy with the right person, and once you've found a partner, you will have sex many, many more times than required to have a family, just for the fun of it.

Contents

Teenage boys guide to sexuality

Your *cock*

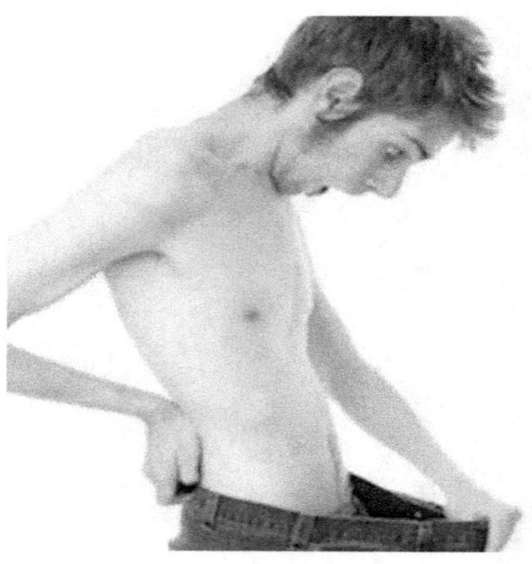

Your *dick* is amazing, and you have every right to love it and enjoy it. Guys are born with their very own shape-shifter, I mean, how

cool is that?

Sometimes, you may find that it shape-shifts (you catch a *boner*) for no reason at all and at inopportune moments and this may feel embarrassing. There's no need for embarrassment as it's normal, and besides, nobody looks that closely; it probably won't even be noticed. If you do feel conspicuous, sit down for a few minutes and wait for it to pass.

80's comedian Billy Connolly says that a penis can't tell the difference between a woman and a bumpy bus ride, so even old guys sometimes have this problem :/

You'll most likely get hard while you sleep and often wake up with a *boner*. This is a normal part of your body's functioning and we fondly call this our *morning wood.*

You've probably wondered how your *meat*

stick matches up to other boys; does it look different, is it too small or brown or bent? Why do I have more skin than the other boys in the locker room, or less? Am I *normal*?

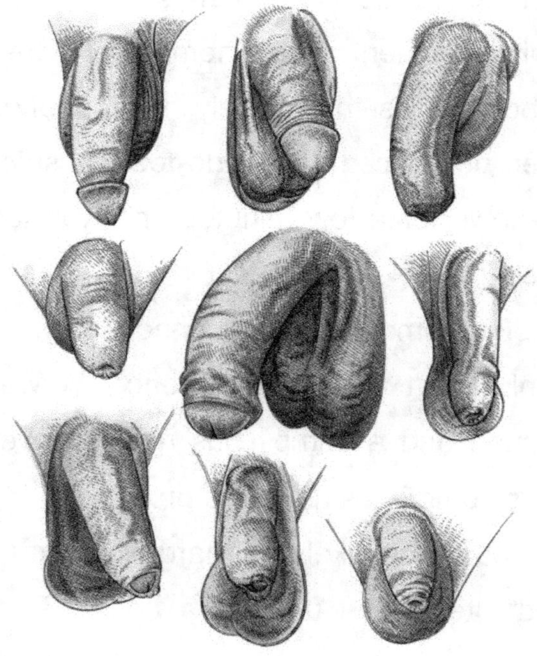

These are just a few variations, but there are many others.

Just like the rest of our bodies, our faces, lips, eyes, etc, unless you have a medical condition that was detected at birth, your penis is normal no matter what it looks like.

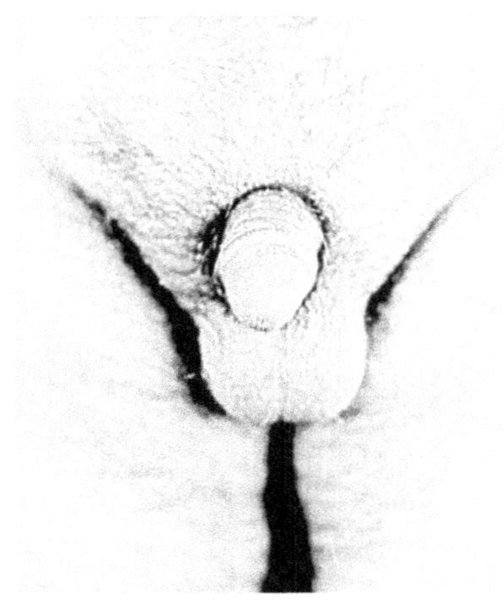

Circumcised, or *cut* penis, sitting atop the balls

There are dozens of variations, from show-ers (long when flaccid) to growers (short when flaccid but grow just as big as the show-ers), to straight, to bent, to thick, to thin, to circumcised to not.

Some soft *willies* sit high above the balls, while others hang down over them.

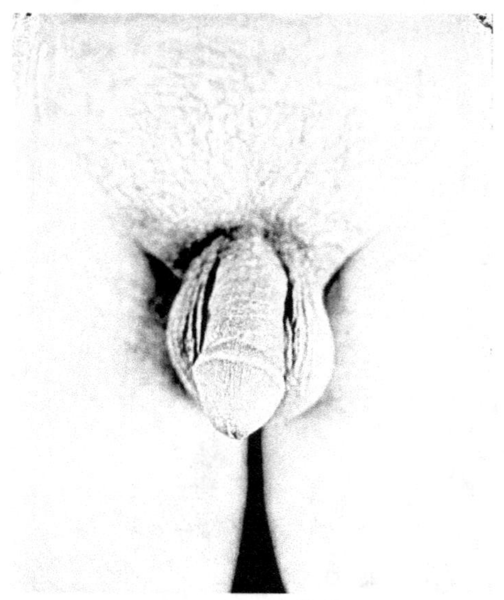

Another circumcised cock, hanging over the balls

Some *boners* are arrow straight while others bend to the side, or up or down. It may be lighter in colour than the rest of your body, or darker, or even change colour along the shaft, especially if you are circumcised. You might have a prominent vein on the surface of your cock or you may have no visible veins at all.

Are you *cut*? This is another term for circumcised, and as a young boy, I had no idea if I was or wasn't, never having seen another penis to compare against.

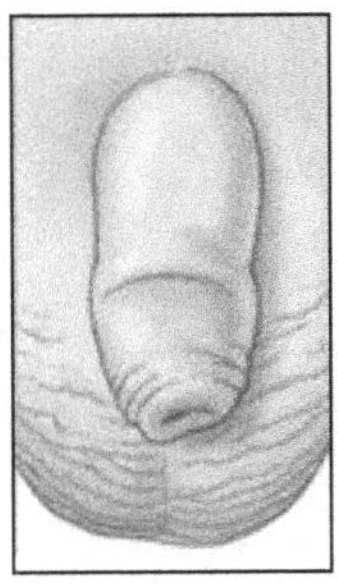

Natural penis

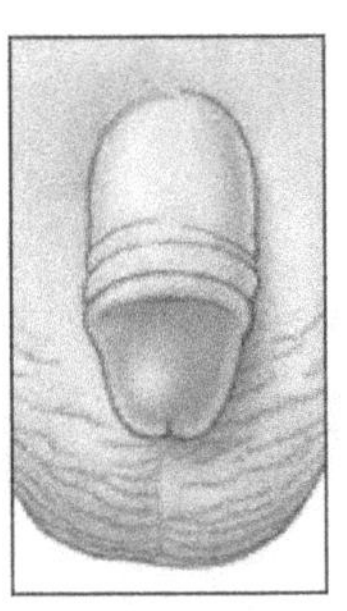

Circumcised penis

© Healthwise, Incorporated

Circumcision is the removal of the

foreskin, which is a tube of skin that slips over the tip of the penis. Uncut boys need to pull their foreskins back and wash thoroughly around the tip to avoid bad smells and possible infection.

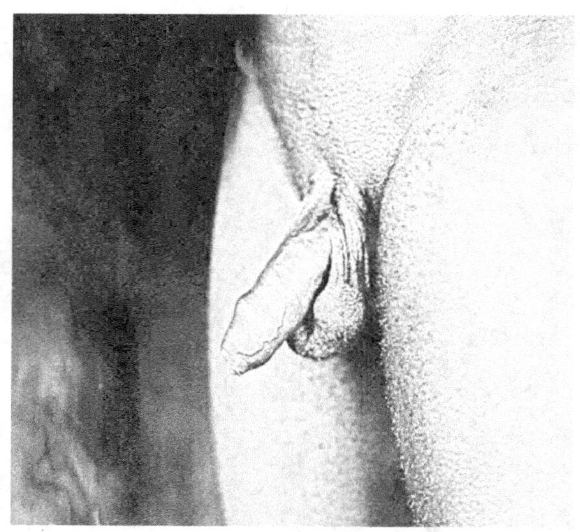

Short foreskin, visible vein

The tip of the dick is called the glans which is a head that looks like a little helmet. It has a cleft on the underside where a lot of nerves converge making it a very sensitive area, and a hole in the middle to pee and cum out of.

If the head is always visible, then you are most likely cut. Even circumcisions have different appearances, with a tight circumcision meaning that there is no loose

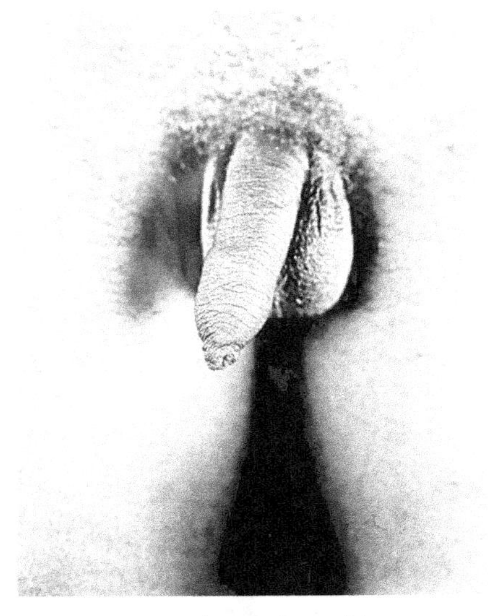

Long foreskin

skin that ever touches the tip, and a loose circumcision where sometimes the base of the tip might have some skin covering it.

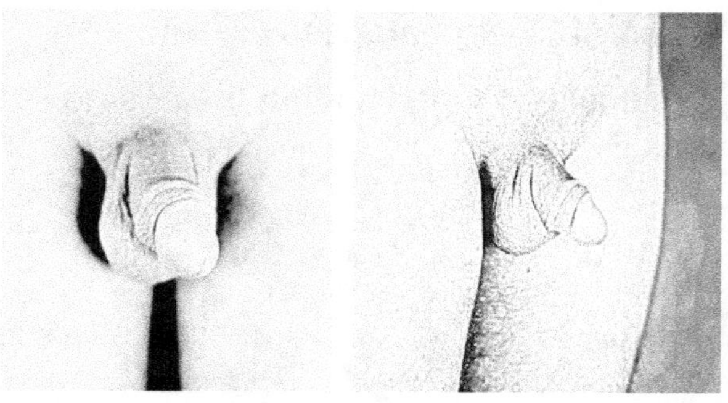

All normal!

There are many reasons for boys being cut. It may be for religious or cultural reasons (Jews, Muslims, some Christians, many Americans, Xhosas), health reasons and the prevention of HIV, or simply a personal preference of the parents, or the boy himself when he is older.

Sometimes, as guys enter their teens, their foreskin may not be loose enough when they get hard which causes a fair amount of pain, and a circumcision or loosening of the foreskin is required. If it's painful to have an erection, speak to your doctor.

It was found in a study that a lot of men who experienced tight foreskins simply did not *jack off* enough, and when encouraged to do so more often, the foreskin loosened up in a few weeks. (Men's health Q&A)

When erect, some foreskins automatically pull back from the head while others only pull back when engaged in actual fucking, or pulled back by hand. The single concern for a foreskin that does not pull back fully, if there is no pain, is cleanliness and a higher likelihood of infection.

An uncut *hard-on* looks pretty much the same as a cut one, with just a bit more play on the skin surrounding the shaft. Some people think a cut penis looks nicer, others think an uncut cock looks nicer. Some think sex is better if you have a foreskin, others disagree. All just about personal preference.

If you are cut, you may be able to see a scar and a change of colour on your shaft where the foreskin was removed.

Okay, I know you want to know about size, and you've been very patient so far.

If you've measured your boner, don't feel embarrassed, just about every guy alive has. Just make sure you're doing it correctly, along the top or side from where it joins your body to the hole at the tip. You know what I'm about to say next; there is no *normal;* hard-ons come in all sizes from just a few inches to giant monsters that make it difficult to have sex as it's too painful for the partner.

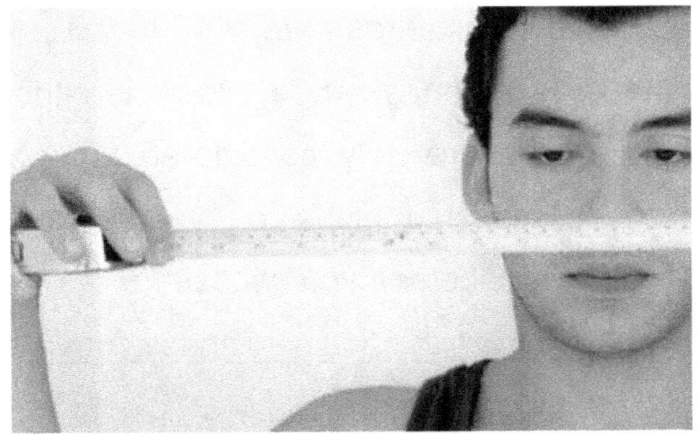

Before I tell you what the average cock size is, let me tell you that size is not related to the amount of pleasure you can give a partner. While having a bigger than average *woody* might be great for the ego, it doesn't necessarily mean better equipped to satisfy a girlfriend/boyfriend. An attentive, caring lover will do better than one who relies solely on the fact that he has a big *knob*.

Okay, here it is. An average size *dong* is 6 to 10 centimetres when soft (2.3" to 3.9") and 12 to 16 centimetres hard (4.7" to 6.3"). Let's call it 14cm on average. Penis lengthening procedures are only considered for *boners* 7cm or less, so if this *is* you, you can discuss it with your doctor *if you choose to.*

https://www.medicalnewstoday.com/articles/271647.php

Your balls will naturally become hairy as you mature, and hair will even grow along the underside of your cock to some extent. As we get older, some guys choose to shave completely or to trim neatly with a pair of scissors or electric shaver. There is a benefit to this as it makes your *junk* easier to keep clean and keep it smelling fresh.

The reason is that all this hair traps sweat

which can become a bit smelly and require more frequent washing. Powdering your balls after you shower will also help keep them fresh and stop them itching in the heat.

If you sometimes find a white substance on your dick, it is normal and has a name: smegma. It is not dangerous and does not mean you have any sort of disease or infection. Washing your cock every day with soap and water will prevent smegma from building up, which you want to do, as if it builds up for a long period of time, the bacteria contained in it may cause irritation or infection. Also, it doesn't smell very nice.

Masturbation

Masturbation is making a fist around your cock and rubbing up and down until you cum.

I know I said I wasn't going to use clinical terms, but masturbation is the parent of so many other phrases that refer to the same thing. Some of these terms have no logical explanation, some are funny, some are graphic. *Choking the chicken*, for example, is visual and funny.

Here are a few more:

Wanking, jerking off, jacking off, walking

the dog, spanking the monkey, flogging the dolphin, Mrs Palmer and her five daughters, polishing the bishop. There are hundreds of terms for it which just goes to show how much time guys spend thinking about it.

A lot of people believe, incorrectly, that the bible says jerking off is a sin. That's just stupid when there isn't a healthy male alive who doesn't do it.

The story of Onan is the one people use to "prove" this fact, but they are not quoting it in its entire context.

Onan is said to have sinned by *spilling his seed upon the ground*, which gives us another common word for masturbation, which is *onanism*. Many tight-lipped finger-pointers insist that this is a direct condemnation of *choking the chicken*. When you put this in its proper context, it's not

Onan's *jerking off* that was sinful, but his belligerent defiance of God's will. God had commanded Onan to impregnate his dead brother's wife to continue the familial line, but Onan deliberately chose to *wank* rather than perform this duty, thus making his defiance of God obvious. *That* was the sin, not masturbation.

For many boys from religious backgrounds, their faith and belief in the teachings cause countless years of shame and self-loathing as they find themselves "sinning" again and again, by doing things that are completely normal and in our nature as human males.

Nature designed our bodies to be enjoyed in so many ways; delicious food, beautiful views, back tickles, a wonderful fragrance, and sexual pleasure, on our own or with a partner.

Homosexuality, too, is perfectly normal and healthy; we don't get to choose if we want to be straight or gay, nature decides this for us.

As I said earlier, sex is *not* primarily for reproduction. It is primarily for enjoyment and good health, as sex not only feels good in the moment but leaves you feeling happy and content as a sexual being, plus is a great form of exercise. Sex, more so than other forms of exercise, releases endorphins which make your body feel energised and alive.

The fact that sex makes us feel attractive and appreciated as well is another boost for our self-esteem and our mental well-being.

So, who wanks? Is it harmful? What's its

purpose?

Pretty much all males do it throughout their lives, even after they are married. For some, a minority, it happens infrequently, whilst for many, it happens on a regular basis.

Both are normal, there is no right or wrong. Several times a day is normal for some, whilst once a month is normal for others. The important thing to realise is that no matter how frequently you are *flogging the dolphin*, you are not an anomaly and your friends are probably doing it just as often and having the same worries as you.

It doesn't stop when you get older, grown ass men of 50, 60, 80 even, still *jerk off*, just not as frequently as when they were younger.

Not only is *wanking* normal and nothing to be ashamed of, it is a healthy way for boys to learn about their bodies and prepare for a time when they will be having sex with another person. It helps you learn what feels good and what doesn't, what hurts and what works.

Shooting a load can help you relax if you are feeling stressed, or to fall asleep if your mind is full of noise. And hey, sometimes, it just feels good so why not?

Everybody wanks differently. Many uncut guys rub the shaft, which causes the foreskin to move back and forth over the head. Some guys prefer to focus mostly on the head while others will focus on the shaft more.

Jerking off does feel different to sex as the stimulation is more focused on the part of your dick that works best for you.

With sex, the sensation is more from the pressure around your shaft which is less intense, and so will usually take longer.

Sex is a holistic experience, however, involving the entire body, and caressing and exploring your partner's body with your hands and tongue will add to your enjoyment of the experience and boost your horniness, so it doesn't matter that the penis isn't getting first-hand stimulation, so to speak.

Horny means in the mood to have sex, feeling horny.

Avoid wanking with soap as it can sting and cause inflammation if it enters the tip. Rather use baby oil or buy lubrication from any supermarket. Not only will this stop you from having a chaffed willy, it also feels a lot nicer than a dry hand.

If you want to know more about wanking, visit http://www.healthystrokes.com/young.html

Your *balls*

Your *balls* hang under your dick and may hardly be noticeable until your testicles drop into the scrotum, or *ball bag,* which happens in early puberty. The external sack that hangs down is your scrotum which is split in two by a thin seam, and if you gently squeeze it you'll feel an oval-shaped object inside each one; these are your actual testicles.

Feeling the shape of your testicles is actually a very important part of remaining healthy. You should check them regularly, especially when you are older, as any change in their shape may indicate a medical problem such as cancer. If you find that your testicles have a bump on them or change shape, contact your doctor for a check-up to be safe.

Getting enjoyment from stroking or squeezing your balls, or tugging on them, is also a normal form of stimulation.

The area between the underside of your balls and your arsehole is called the perineum and caressing this bit of skin is also pleasurable.

Balls, too, differ from guy to guy; some have tight *nut sacks* with little sway and others have balls that hang down way lower than their dicks, which can be uncomfortable if venturing out the house without underwear (going *commando*), or playing sports. Some have smaller balls and others have big, full-looking *ball sacks*.

You'll notice your *scrote* (short for scrotum) hangs lower when it is hot, or you are in a hot bath, and tightens up in the cold, all for the single purpose of ensuring the health of your sperm-guys.

On many males, one testicle hangs lower than the other, the left being more common, oddly enough.

The skin itself is very pliable and may also change texture depending on the temperature, or if you are hard or soft. At times your ball bag may be completely wrinkled and at others, it may be quite smooth or have what appears to be goosebumps.

It may be browner or pinker than the rest of your body and sometimes veins may be noticeable. It is very similar to elbow skin, where pliability is also important. Which reminds me of a joke:

An angel comes up to God and says, "Dude, we've got all this left-over elbow skin, what should we do with it?"

And God replies, "Why don't we make little bags for them to keep their balls in?"

Ejaculation

Medically known as ejaculation, *cumming* is synonymous with orgasm in guys and is when semen, or *cum,* is shot out of the cock at speeds of up to 50km/h (31 mph).

Again, the way we cum is different for different people, and some will shoot a fair distance, maybe hitting themselves in the eye, while others tend more to bubble and dribble.

A lot of guys cum in their sleep and all you'll know about it is when you wake up sticky. This is called a *wet dream* or nocturnal emission and is your body's way of keeping the sperm in your balls young and fresh.

The amount of *cock-snot* ejected is generally about a teaspoon or two, but this varies with the intensity of the orgasm and the length of time since you last came. It ejaculates in "pulses", on average about 7 to 10 spurts an orgasm, lasting between 10 and 30 seconds, more if you're lucky.

A lot of guys, but not all, experience *pre-cum*, which is a translucent fluid that leaks from your dick throughout the stimulation leading to *climax*. Even though pre-cum generally contains very little actual sperm, it may still be enough to cause pregnancy, so thinking it is safe to *shag* if you pull out before you cum is not a gamble you should ever take. (Condoms!)

Thirty years ago, the pope decreed that using a condom was a sin, and so many Catholics used this method of contraception, earning it the title, *The Catholic Method.* (Have you seen how large Catholic families from that generation are?!)

If you've tasted your own cum, again, nothing that a lot of guys haven't done before you. In fact, maybe it's only fair that you do if you expect somebody else to taste it someday!

The taste varies based on a few things like diet, exercise and smoking. A high protein diet and smoking makes for a stronger, more pungent taste, while a lot of water and fruit makes it less of an assault on the tongue.

Semen is completely safe to swallow as it consists primarily of vitamins, calcium, protein, zinc and so on.

If you cum regularly, your semen will probably appear more translucent than if you abstain for a while, in which case it may have quite a thick, gloppy look to it. The smell may also be more intense the longer you abstain and the colour slightly more yellowish.

Sexual orientation

Even if you know you are straight, I suggest you read this section to understand a little more about gay guys.

It used to be a simplified portrayal by society that you were either attracted to girls or boys. I say *portrayal* because the following sexual identities have always existed, but it's only in recent times that society has started to give them a voice.

Now we have heterosexual, homosexual, pansexual, bisexual, asexual, gender-fluid, trans and a whole bunch more.

Commonly known, heterosexuals (straights) are attracted to the opposite sex, while homosexuals (gays and lesbians) are attracted to the same sex.

Trans, or *transgender,* are people whose intrinsic sense of identity does not coincide with the gender that they were born with. For example, a person who was born as a male but for all intents and purposes, mentally and emotionally, identifies internally as female.

Bisexual means that you are physically attracted to both men and women who identify themselves according to their birth gender, i.e. not as trans.

Pansexual refers to those who are attracted to anybody, regardless of gender or gender identity, so men, women and trans people. They are attracted to a person's aura, energy and personality.

Gender-fluid denotes those who do not identify themselves as belonging to one or the other of the genders.

Asexual are those who are without sexual feelings or urges, who live contentedly without sex. This is not common, but if you feel this way, realise that it is totally acceptable and normal.

What does it mean? It means you are free to be whomever nature intended, no matter how you identify yourself sexually or who you find yourself attracted to, without guilt or shame. For simplicity, and so as not to boggle my own brain, I'm going to stick with gay and straight, which basically means that you will be attracted to one or other of the genders.

For about 95% of guys it's simple; they think about boobs, like a *lot*, they like girls in bikinis, they fantasize about girls when they *beat the meat* and they have a healthy preoccupation with the opposite sex.

Of the 5% who don't fit the heterosexual mould, it's only the same for a handful of them; they know from a young age that they look at guys and not girls, they like a firm butt on a guy and a tight six-pack and they have a healthy preoccupation with the same sex. They understand their sexual orientation and don't feel the need to agonise over it.

But for many, it's far more complicated. Maybe a failed sexual encounter with a girl has left you wondering why you couldn't get it up. *Am I gay?*

Well, probably not. Our first time is scary, and sometimes our nerves get the better of us, and that's all it is. Sometimes we just develop later than other guys and don't find a particular fascination with boobs until our late teens.

But if you're jerking off to pictures of Justin Bieber skinny dipping, well in that case, yes, you might be gay (or bi.)

Too many gay guys vehemently refuse to accept that it might be true, because our parents, teachers, preachers, friends, relatives teach us that there is something perverted or depraved about homosexuality. If not with outright condemnation then with subtle clues, such as homophobic jokes or derisive comments. If you are gay, it might take months, or it might take years to reconcile yourself with the truth.

If you are in this minority, things could be tough. Your choices are either to be true to yourself and risk ostracization or betray yourself and maintain the status quo.

Sometimes, coming out is as bad as we anticipate, sometimes the people who love us will surprise us. You'd be gobsmacked at how many parents and friends already know without you having to tell them, sometimes even before you do.

Nothing shows you who your true friends are better than coming out.

Unfortunately, in some cultures it is taboo, which of course doesn't stop gay people being born, it just forces them to live dual lives, a public persona and a private one. Even in countries where homosexuality carries the penalty of death, gay people find it practically impossible to suppress their true natures. And they tell us it's a choice?

I can't tell you how to come out, or even if coming out is the right thing for you to do, but I can tell you something that only a gay person can understand. It's *not* a choice to be gay. Considering the persecution that gay people are exposed to the world over, who in their right mind would be gay if they had a choice not to be? Remember this argument if anybody ever suggests otherwise.

All you need to know is that you are gay by *design*, not by choice, and anybody who rejects you on that basis might just as well reject you for being blond/ginger/brunette/tall/short or any other facet that you have no control over. You are perfect in nature's grand scheme and owe no apology for who you are, have nothing to be ashamed of or embarrassed about.

This is the basis of *gay pride*, which is *not* about being proud that we're gay (as so many heterosexuals think), but about being proud to have found the courage to stand up and be ourselves in the face of adversity. Gay pride parades are about saying, "this is me, take it or leave it."

Sex is a responsibility

Don't rush it.

Sex is great, but along with it comes complicated, confusing emotions and repercussions when you are young. And it doesn't really get a whole lot simpler when you're older, either.

If you are *straight*, it's important to realise this nasty trick that nature plays on us: guys and girls have different expectations of losing their virginity. Guys are thinking *fuck* and *get laid,* while for girls it's more *making love*. For us, it's more focused on the physical, while girls have a stronger coupling between the physical and emotional. What is just a lay to you might be an intimate relationship to her. You need to understand and respect that.

Don't take this step lightly. Don't pressure another person to have sex. Remember that sex is not just a physical act; it's a mingling of auras, a union of souls that has meaning and will have an impact on each of you. Are you mature enough to deal with the emotions of revealing your body and soul to another person? How will you feel about that person tomorrow?

When you are ready, and your girlfriend/boyfriend is ready, *use a condom*. I know, nothing new there.

But seriously, straight guys: picture what your life would be like a year from now with a baby in it. And no, **it is not** just the girl's problem. When you have sex with someone you are accepting an unspoken contract between you, which means *joint* responsibility for your decision and the consequences.

And gay guys? Sure, no pregnancy, but you *and* the straight boys stand the risk of HIV, gonorrhoea, syphilis and a bunch of other *horrible* diseases that could make big ugly boils appear on your balls, or your cock to emit a foul-smelling yellow goo. Crabs on your balls are also no fun at all.

It's your *life*. <u>Just don't do it.</u>

Other questions?

If you have any questions that were not answered in this booklet, email me at <u>guytoguy@copyediting.co.nz</u> and I will do my best to answer them. Note that any questions you ask may be published in future editions, but your personal details will not be revealed.

Remember, your body is yours to enjoy and if what you are doing is not harmful to yourself or any other person or animal, it's okay to be doing it, and has been done by millions of guys before you. But remember, everything in moderation. If you find yourself becoming obsessed with sex/porn/wanking or are in doubt about any other aspect of sex, ask your doctor for advice. They are trained professionals who have heard it all before and will advise without judgement.

And always be safe.

Your go-to-guy,

Tim

Teenage boys guide to sexuality